Irving's
Anatomy
Mnemonics

Alastair G Smith
LRCP and S (Edin)
Senior Demonstrator in Anatomy,
Surgeon's Hall, Edinburgh

FOURTH EDITION

CHURCHILL LIVINGSTONE
EDINBURGH LONDON AND NEW YORK

CHURCHILL LIVINGSTONE
Medical Division of Longman Group UK Limited

Distributed in the United States of America
by Churchill Livingstone Inc., 1560 Broadway,
New York, N.Y. 10036 and by associated
companies branches and representatives throughout
the world.

Fourth Edition
    Twenty-fourth reprint 1985
    Twenty-fifth reprint 1988
    Twenty-sixth reprint 1989
    Twenty-seventh reprint 1990
    Twenty-eighth reprint 1991

ISBN 0-443-00253-3

Produced by Longman Group (FE) Ltd
Printed in Hong Kong

Preface

To the simple-minded, to the crammers for exams, and to those whose stumbling feet find the Anatomical Pathway difficult, this little book is offered in the hope rather than the belief that they may find some help from it.

Surgeons' Hall,   AGS
Edinburgh, October, 1939.

ARTERIAL SYSTEM.

AORTA is subdivided into:—

(1) Ascending Aorta.

Begins from left ventricle opposite 3rd costal cartilage at left margin of sternum.

Ends opposite 2nd right costal cartilage at right margin of sternum.

Branches:

Right and left coronary.

(2) Arch of Aorta.

Begins opposite 2nd right costal cartilage.

Ends at left side of lower border of 4th thoracic vertebra.

Branches:

(1) Innominate;
(2) Left common carotid;
(3) Left subclavian.

Relations :

5 things post. and to right.

(1) Trachea ;
(2) Oesophagus ;
(3) Left recurrent N. ;
(4) Thoracic duct ;
(5) Vertebral cloumn.

5 things ant. and to left.

(1) Lung and pleura ;
(2) Left phrenic ;
(3) Left vagus ;
(4) Cardiac nerves ;
(5) Superior intercostal vein.

5 things below.

(1) Left bronchus ;
(2) Right pulmonary artery ;
(3) Lig. arteriosum ;
(4) Left recurrent laryngeal nerve ;
(5) Superficial cardiac plexus.

5 things above.

(1) Left common carotid ;
(2) Left subclavian ;
(3) Innominate ;
(4) Thymus ;
(5) Left innominate vein.

(3) Descending Thoracic Aorta:

Begins at left side of lower border of 4th thoracic vertebra.

Ends at lower border of 12th dorsal vertebra by becoming abdominal aorta.

Branches:

9 Aortic intercostals;
4 Oesophageal;
3 Bronchial;
2 Diaphragmatic.
Mediastinal, pericardial and subcostal.

Relations:

	Anterior.		*Right.*
L.	Root of left lung.	**R.**	Right lung and pleura.
O.	Oesophagus.	**O.**	Oesophagus.
A.	Left atrium.	**A.**	Vena azygos.
D.	Diaphragm.	**D.**	Thoracic duct and dorsal vertebrae.

Left.	*Posterior.*
HE. Hemiazygos veins.	**H.** Hemiazygos vein.
L. Left lung.	**I.** Intercostal arteries.
P. Pleura.	**L.** Longitudinal ligament and vertebral column.
S. Splanchnic N.	**L.** Left lung and pleura.

(4) Abdominal Aorta:

Begins at lower margin of 12th thoracic vertebra.
Ends at lower margin of 4th lumbar vertebra by sub-dividing into two common iliacs.

Branches :

Please,	Phrenics.
Can	Coeliac artery.
Soft	Middle suprarenal.
Soap	Superior mesenteric.
Remove	Renal.
Tint	Testicular.
In	Inferior mesenteric.
Ladies'	Lumbar.
Stockings ?	Middle sacral.

Relations :

	Anterior.	Posterior.
Put	Coeliac and aortic plexuses.	**3 Ls:** Lumbar vertebrae. Longitudinal ligament 3rd and 4th left lumbar veins.
Pancreas	Body and uncinate process of pancreas.	
Spleen	Splenic vein.	
Mesentery	Superior mesenteric artery.	
Right	Left renal vein.	
Down	3rd part of duodenum.	
In	Inferior mesenteric artery.	
My	Root of mesentery	
Paper	Peritoneum.	
Immediately.	Small intestine.	

	Right.		*Left.*
Remember	Right crus.	**Universities**	Left ureter.
Inferior	Inferior vena cava.	**Make**	Inferior mesenteric vein.
Vena	Vena azygos.	**Students**	Sympathetic trunk.
Cava.	Cisterna chyli.	**Sorrowfully**	Small intestine.
		Pursue	Peritoneum.
		Dull	Terminal part of duodenum.
		Courses.	Left crus.

Innominate Artery:

Begins opposite centre of manubrium from aortic arch.

Ends behind upper part of sternoclavicular joint by dividing into right common carotid and right subclavian.

Relations :

	Anterior.	*Right.*	*Posterior.*	*Left.*
Travelling	Thymus.			
L.	Left innominate vein.			
M.	Manubrium.			
S.	Sternoclavicular joint. Sternohyoid. Sternothyroid.			
Is		Right innominate vein. Superior vena cava.		
Take			Trachea.	
Less			Lung and pleura.	
Money.			Longus cervicis muscle.	
Considered				Left common carotid.
To				Trachea.

NOTES

Common Carotid Artery:

Begins on right side from bifurcation of innominate behind sterno-clavicular joint on left side from aortic arch.

Ends by subdividing into external and internal carotids at upper border of thyroid cartilage opposite 3rd cervical inter-vertebral disc.

Relations in Neck:

Superficial.

1 Artery—
  Sternomastoid artery from the superior thyroid.

2 Nerves—
  (1) Descendens hypoglossi;
  (2) Ansa hypoglossi.

3 Veins—
  (1) Internal jugular;
  (2) Anterior jugular;
  (3) Middle thyroid.

Deep.

1 Structure—
  Thoracic duct.

2 Muscles—
  (1) Longus cervicis;
  (2) Longus capitis.

3 Arteries—
  (1) Subclavian;
  (2) Vertebral;
  (3) Inferior thyroid.

4 Muscles—
(1) Sternomastoid;
(2) Sternohyoid;
(3) Sternothyroid;
(4) Omohyoid.

5 Structures—
(1) Skin;
(2) Superficial fascia;
(3) Platysma;
(4) Deep fascia;
(5) Thyroid body.

Medial.

6 Structures—
(1) Larynx;
(2) Trachea;
(3) Pharynx;
(4) Oesophagus; [nerve;
(5) Recurrent laryngeal
(6) Thyroid body.

4 Nerves—
(1) Sympathetic trunk;
(2) Middle cervical gan-
glion;
(3) Vagus;
(4) Recurrent laryngeal
nerves.

Lateral.

(1) Internal jugular;
(2) Vagus;
(3) Apex of lung and pleura.

External Carotid Artery:

Begins from bifurcation of common carotid at upper border of thyroid cartilage opposite 3rd cervical intervertebral disc.

Ends opposite the neck of the condyle of the mandible by subdivision into superficial temporal and maxillary.

Relations :

Superficial.

1 Structure—
   The parotid gland which envelops the artery.

2 Nerves—
   (1) Facial ;
   (2) Hypoglossal.

3 Muscles—
   (1) Sternomastoid ;
   (2) Post belly of digastric ;
   (3) Stylohyoid.

Deep.

1 Bone—
   Styloid process.

2 Arteries—
   (1) Ascending pharyngeal ;
   (2) Internal carotid.

3 Muscles—
   (1) Styloglossus ;
   (2) Stylopharyngeus ;
   (3) Constrictors of pharynx.

4 Veins—	4 Nerves—
(1) Superior thyroid;	(1) Glossopharyngeal nerve;
(2) Lingual;	(2) Pharyngeal branch of vagus;
(3) Common facial;	(3) Internal laryngeal nerve;
(4) Post facial.	(4) External laryngeal nerve.

Branches :

Sweet	Superior thyroid.
Little	Lingual.
Flappers	Facial.
Occupy	Occipital.
Positions	Post auricular.
As	Ascending pharyngeal.
Stenographers	Superficial temporal.
Mainly.	Maxillary.

B

Superior Thyroid:

Begins from external carotid close to its origin.

Ends by distribution to the anterior surface of thyroid body in its proximal two-thirds.

Branches:

May	Muscular.
I	Infrahyoid.
Softly	Superior laryngeal.
Squeeze	Sternomastoid.
Charlie's	Cricothyroid.
Girl?	Glandular.

Lingual Artery:

Begins from external carotid opposite the tip of the greater cornu of hyoid bone.

Ends as profunda linguae to tip of tongue.

Relations :

Superficial.	Deep.
6 Structures—	**3** Structures—
1 Duct—	(1) Middle constrictor ;
Submandibular duct.	(2) Genioglossus ;
2 Nerves—	(3) Stylohyoid lig.
(1) Hypoglossal ;	
(2) Lingual.	
3 Muscles—	
(1) Digastric and stylo-hyoid ;	
(2) Hyoglossus ;	
(3) Mylohyoid.	

Branches :

Sing. Suprahyoid.
Daddy. Dorsalis linguae.
Sing. Sublingual.

Facial Artery:

Origin from external carotid half an inch above tip of greater cornu of hyoid.

Ends at medial canthus.

Branches :

And	Ascending palatine.
Tonsils	Tonsillar.
Go	Glandular.
Septic	Submental.
In	Inferior labial.
Some	Superior labial.
Little	Lateral nasal.
Mouths.	Muscular.

Maxillary Artery:

Begins opposite the neck of the condyle of the mandible from the bifurcation of the external carotid.

Ends in the pterygo-palatine fossa by subdivision into its terminal branches.

Course is subdivided into three parts by the lateral pterygoid

Branches :

All	Auricular.	From 1st part— proximal to lateral pterygoid.
Try	Tympanic.	
My	Middle meningeal.	
Ample	Accessory meningeal.	
Instructions	Inferior dental.	
To	Deep temporal.	From 2nd part— superficial to lateral pterygoid.
Produce	Pterygoid.	
Magnificent	Masseteric.	
Blossoms	Buccinator.	
Published	Post superior dental	From 3rd part— in the pterygo-palatine fossa.
In	Infraorbital.	
A	Artery of the pterygoid canal.	
Pamphlet	Palatine.	
Price	Pharyngeal.	
Sixpence.	Sphenopalatine.	

Internal Carotid Artery:

Begins from bifurcation of common carotid at upper border of thyroid cartilage opposite 3rd cervical intervertebral disc.

Ends at anterior perforated substance by subdividing into anterior and middle cerebrals.

Branches:

Carotid	Carotico-tympanic.
Passes	Pterygoid.
Cautiously	Cavernous.
Down	Dural.
Past	Pituitary.
Ganglion.	Ganglionic (trigeminal ganglion).
Ophthalmic	Ophthalmic.
Presently	Posterior-communicating.
Courses	Choroidal.
Anteriorly	Anterior cerebral.
Mainly.	Middle cerebral.

Ophthalmic Artery:

Begins from internal carotid after perforation of dura on medial side of anterior clinoid process.

Ends at anterior part of orbit by subdivision into dorsal nasal and supratrochlear.

Branches :

Lady	Lachrymal.
Students	Supraorbital.
Must	Meningeal.
Remember	Arteria retinae centralis.
College	Ciliary—long and short posterior.
Examiners	Anterior and posterior ethmoidal.
Plough	Medial palpebral.
Some	Supratrochlear.
Duffers.	Dorsal nasal.

Subclavian Artery:

Begins (1) Left side—from aortic arch about half an inch below the sternoclavicular joint; (2) Right side—from bifurcation of the innominate at the sternoclavicular joint.

Ends on both sides at the lateral border of the first rib by becoming the axillary artery.

Course is subdivided into three parts by the scalenus anterior muscle.

Relations—1st Part :

Anterior :

3 Muscles—Sternomastoid, sternohyoid, sternothyroid.

3 Veins—Internal jugular, anterior jugular, and vertebral.

3 Nerves—Phrenic, vagus, and cardiac.

6 Structures—Skin, superior fascia, platysma, deep fascia, common carotid, thoracic duct or right lymph duct.

Posterior :

Lung and pleura, thoracic duct or right lymph duct, longus cervicis, with oesophagus extra on left side and recurrent laryngeal nerve on right.

Relations—3rd Part :

1 Relations below :
   1st rib.

2 Relations above :
   Transverse cervical artery
   lowest trunk of brachial plexus.

3 Relations posterior :
   Lung and pleura
   scalenus medius
   lowest trunk of brachial plexus.

5 Sets of relations anterior :

1 Bone—Clavicle.

2 Muscles—Platysma and subclavius.

3 Nerves—Nerve to subclavius, intermediate and lateral
   supraclavicular nerves.

4 Veins—External jugular, anterior jugular, transverse
   cervical, and suprascapular.

5 Structures—Skin, superficial fascia, deep fascia, pre-
   vertebral fascia, and the suprascapular artery.

Branches :

Vertebrae	Vertebral.
Make	Internal mammary.
The	Thyrocervical trunk. $\begin{cases} \text{Inferior thyroid.} \\ \text{Transverse cervical.} \\ \text{Suprascapular.} \end{cases}$
Column.	Costocervical trunk. $\begin{cases} \text{Superior intercostal.} \\ \text{Deep cervical.} \end{cases}$

Vertebral Artery:

Begins from 1st part of subclavian one half inch medial to scalenus anterior.

Ends at lower border of pons by joining its fellow to form basilar artery.

Branches :

Muscular	Muscular.
S.	Spinal.
P.	Posterior inferior cerebellar.
A.	Anastomotic.
S.	Spinal (anterior, posterior).
M.	Meningeal and medullary.

Internal Mammary Artery:

Begins from lower border of 1st part of subclavian at the medial edge of scalenus anterior.

Ends at 6th intercostal space by subdivision into superior epigastric and musculo-phrenic.

Relations:

Anterior:

Phrenic	Phrenic.
Nerve	Internal intercostal nerves.
Crosses	Costal cartilages.
Internal mammary	Internal intercostal muscles.
In	Internal jugular vein.
Contact.	Clavicle.

Posterior.

P. Pleura.

S. Sternocostalis.

Branches:

An	Anterior intercostals.
M.P.	Mediastinal and pericardio-phrenic.
P.Ms.	Perforating, musculo-phrenic and superior epigastric.

Axillary Artery:

Begins as the continuation of the subclavian at the lateral border of the 1st rib.

Ends by changing its name to brachial at the distal edge of the teres major.

Course is subdivided into **3 parts** by the pectoralis minor muscle.

Branches :

- **S.** Superior thoracic—1ST PART.
- **A.** Acromio-thoracic. } 2ND PART.
- **L.** Lateral thoracic.
- **S.** Subscapular. } 3RD PART.
- **A.** Anterior humeral circumflex.
- **P.** Posterior humeral circumflex.

Relations—1st Part :

Anterior.

- **S.** Middle supraclavicular nerves.
- **C.** Cephalic vein and clavi-pectoral fascia.
- **A.** Acromio-thoracic artery.
- **L.** Lateral pectoral nerve.
- **P.** Pectoralis major.

Posterior.

- **P.** Medial pectoral nerve.
- **R.** 2nd rib.
- **I.** 1st intercostal space.
- **S.** Nerve to serratus anterior.
- **M.** Medial cord.
- **S.** Serratus anterior.

Anterior.

2 Structures—
  (1) Pectoralis major ;
  (2) Pectoralis minor.

Medial.

2 Structures—
  (1) Axillary vein ;
  (2) Median cord.

Posterior.

2 Structures—
  (1) Subscapularis ;
  (2) Posterior cord.

Lateral.

2 Structures—
  (1) Coracoid process ;
  (2) Lateral cord.

Medial.

Very	Vein.
Many	Medial cutaneous nerve of arm.
Medicals	Medial cutaneous nerve of forearm.
Must	Medial head of median.
Ultimately	Ulnar nerve.
Marry.	Medial vena comes.

Relations—3rd Part :

Anterior.

Some	Skin.
Fascia	Fascia.
Probably	Pectoralis major.
Clothes	Coracobrachialis (overlaps).
Loosely	Lateral vena comes.
Most	Medial head of the median nerve.
Muscles.	Medial cutaneous nerve of forearm.

30

Posterior.		*Lateral.*	
Some	Subscapularis.	Making	Musculo-cutaneous nerve.
Can	Circumflex nerve.	Most	Median nerve.
Retain	Radial nerve.	Confirmed	Coracobrachialis.
Their	Teres major.	Bachelors.	Biceps.
Liberty.	Latissimus dorsi.		

Brachial Artery:

Begins as continuation of axillary artery at distal edge of teres major.

End in cubital fossa opposite neck of radius by subdivision into radial and ulnar arteries.

Branches :

Practice	Profunda brachii.
Urological	Ulnar collateral.
Surgery	Supratrochlear.
Not	Nutrient.
Modern.	Muscular.

Relations :

	Anterior.		Posterior.
Biceps	Biceps.	Triceps	Triceps (long head, medial head).
Muscle	Median nerve.		Insertion of coracobrachialis.
Mainly	Medial cutaneous nerve of forearm.		
Causes	Median cubital vein.	Is	Profunda brachii artery. Brachialis.
Action	Bicipital aponeurosis.	Pierced	Radial nerve.
Flexion	Fascia.	By	Radial nerve.
Supination.	Skin.		

Medial.

Basilic	Basilic vein.
Follows	Deep fascia.
Ulnar	Ulnar nerve.
Margin	Median nerve.
Closely.	Medial cutaneous nerve of forearm.

Radial Artery:

Begins from bifurcation of brachial artery in the cubital fossa opposite the neck of the radius.

Ends as deep palmar arch by union with deep division of ulnar artery on the radial side of 5th metacarpal bone.

Course is subdivided into 3 parts, viz.:—

(1) From cubital fossa to apex of radial styloid;

(2) From apex of radial styloid to proximal end of 1st metacarpal space on dorsum of hand;

(3) From 1st metacarpal space to radial site of 5th metacarpal base—in palm of hand mainly as deep arch.

Branches :

(1) *In Forearm :*

Member	Muscular.
Royal	Radial recurrent.
College	Anterior radial carpal.
Surgeons.	Superficial palmar.

Post	Posterior radial carpal.
Mortems	Metacarpal.
Denote	Dorsalis pollicis.
Death.	Dorsalis indices.

(3) *In palm:*

Please	Princeps pollicis.
Remember	Radialis indices.
Practice	Perforating (3).
Requires	Recurrent (3).
Patience.	Palmar metacarpals (3).

} From deep arch.

Relations in Forearm:

	Anterior.		*Posterior.*
Surgeons	Skin.	**To**	Tendon of biceps.
Frequently	Fascia.	**Swim**	Supinator.
Clip	Cephalic vein and cutaneous nerves.	**Properly**	Pronator teres.
		Flex	Flexor digitorum sublimus.
Blood	Brachioradialis (overlaps).	**Forearm**	Flexor pollicis longus.
Vessels.	Vena comites (cross branches of).	**Pronate**	Pronator quadratus
		Radius.	Radius.

Ulnar Artery:

Begins from the bifurcation of the brachial in the cubital fossa opposite the neck of the radius.

Ends on the radial side of the pisiform bone by subdivision into superficial and deep divisions.

Branches :

Anatomical	Anterior ulnar recurrent.
Pictures	Posterior ulnar recurrent.
Can	Common interosseous.
Always	Anterior ulnar carpal.
Please.	Posterior ulnar carpal.

Relations :

	Anterior.		_Posterior._
Please	Pronator teres.	**British**	Brachialis.
Fix	Flexa carpi radialis.	**Flag**	Flexor digitorum pro-
My	Median nerve.		fundus.
Fine	Flexor digitorum	**Flies.**	Flexor retinaculum.
	sublimus.		
Pictures	Pelmaris longus.		
Perfectly	Palmar cutaneous		
	branch of ulnar		
	nerve.		

Begins as superficial branch of the ulnar artery at the radial side of the pisiform bone.

Ends a fingers' breadth to the ulnar side of the thumb cleft by completion by anastomosis with the superficial palmar branch of the radial. The middle of the arch cuts the middle of the middle palmar crease.

Branches :

Are four palmar digital arteries to the 2nd, 3rd and 4th clefts and of the ulnar side of the little finger.

Relations :

	Anterior.		*Posterior.*
Pied	Palmaris brevis.	**Men**	Median nerve (digital branches).
Piper	Palmar aponeurosis.	**Often**	Opponens digiti minimi.
Pipes.	Palmar cutaneous branches of median and ulnar nerves.	**Forget**	Flex. digiti minimi.
		Little	Lumbricals,
		Things.	Tendons of flexor sublimus and flexor profundus digitorum.

BRANCHES OF ABDOMINAL AORTA.

Coeliac Artery:

Begins from the abdominal aorta opposite the 1st lumbar vertebra.

Ends behind the lesser sac of peritoneum by subdivision into its three branches.

Course, below the caudate lobe of the liver at the upper border of the pancreas with a crus and a coeliac ganglion on each side.

Branches:

Go	Left gastric.
Straight	Splenic.
Home.	Hepatic.

Splenic Artery:

Begins as a branch of the coeliac artery.

Ends at the hilum of the spleen by subdivision into 5-8 branches.

Branches :

Peter's	Pancreatic.
Spleen	Splenic.
Looks	Left gastro epiploic.
Small.	Short gastric.

Relations :

	Anterior.		*Posterior.*
Lawyers	Lesser sac.	**Legal**	Left crus.
Should	Stomach.	**Candidates**	Left coeliac ganglion.
Practise	Pancreas (upper border).	**Should**	Left suprarenal.
		Know	Left kidney.
Law.	Lieno-renal ligament.	**Latin.**	Lieno-renal ligaments.

Hepatic Artery:

Begins as a branch of the coeliac artery.

Ends at porta hepatis by subdivision into right and left branches.

Branches:

Right	Right gastric.
Gastric	Gastro-duodenal.
Directs	Duodenal.
Round	Right hepatic.
Lesser	Left hepatic.
Curvature.	Cystic (usually from right hepatic).

Superior Mesenteric Artery:

Begins from abdominal aorta in the transpyloric plane opposite the 1st lumbar vertebra, behind the pancreas.

Ends in the right iliac fossa by anastomosing with a branch of the ileo-colic artery.

Branches:

In	Inferior pancreatico duodenal.
Joints	Jejunal.
I	Ileal.
Must	Mid colic.
Remember	Right colic.

Relations :

	Anterior.		Posterior.
Pancreas.	Pancreas.	Ring	Left renal vein.
Sometimes	Splenic vein.	Up	Uncinate process of pancreas.
Marked	Mesentery.	Department	3rd part of duodenum.
Sweetbread.	Small intestine.		Aorta.
		At	Right ureter.
		Royal	Inferior vena cava.
		Infirmary	Testicular vessels.
		To	Genito-femoral nerve.
		Get	
		Physicians.	Psoas.

Renal Arteries:

Begins opposite the 2nd lumbar vertebra from the aorta.

Ends at the hilum of the kidney by subdivision into three primary stems—two in front and one behind the pelvis of the kidney.

Branches :

U. Ureteric.
S. Inferior suprarenal.
R. Renal.

Relations :

Posterior to both.

C. Crus.
P. Psoas.
R. Pelvis renalis.

Right Anterior.

D. Duodenum, 2nd part.
R. Renal veins.
I. Inferior vena cava.

Left Anterior.

R. Renal vein.
I. Inferior mesenteric vein.
P. Pancreas.

Begins from the front of the aorta opposite the 2nd lumbar vertebra.

Ends at the upper pole of the testicle by subdivision into testicular and epididymal branches.

Branches :

C.	Cremasteric.
U.	Ureteric.
T.	Testicular.
E.	Epididymal.

Inferior Mesenteric Artery:

Begins from the front of the aorta opposite the 3rd lumbar vertebra one and a half inches above its bifurcation.

Ends at the middle of the front of the left common iliac artery by becoming the superior rectal.

Relations :

Posterior.

C.   Left common iliac artery.
L.   4th left lumbar vessels.
A.   Aorta.
S.   Sympathetic trunk.
P.   Left psoas.

Branches :

Ushers   Upper left colic.
Like   Lower left colic.
Silence.   Superior rectal.

Common Iliac :

Begins at lower border of left side of 4th lumbar vertebra from bifurcation of aorta.

Ends at lumbo-sacral articulation by subdivision into external

Relations.

Anterior.

Peritoneum.
Intestines.
Sympathetic filaments.
Ureter.
Lower left colic vessels.
Superior rectal vessels.

} Left Common Iliac.

Right Common Iliac. {
Peritoneum
Is
Sometimes
Useful
Lessening
Sepsis.

Posterior.

P. Psoas.
S. Sympathetic trunk.
O. Obturator nerve.
A. Ilio-lumbar artery.
S. Lumbo-sacral trunk.

Plus 5th lumbar vertebra and on right side both common iliac veins.

Internal Iliac:

Begins at lumbo-sacral articulation from bifurcation of common iliac.

Ends at upper margin of great sciatic notch by subdivision into anterior and posterior divisions.

Branches :

Anterior Division.		*Posterior Division.*
Some Superior vesical.		**Such** Superior gluteal.
Inherit Inferior vesical.		**Is** Ilio-lumbar.
Money, Middle rectal.		**Life.** Lateral sacral.
Others Obturator.		
Inherit Internal pudendal.		
Insanity. Inferior gluteal.		

Internal Pudendal Artery.

Branches ;

Rectum	Inferior rectal.
Scrotum	Posterior scrotal.
Bulb	Artery of bulb.
Are Pudendal.	Arteries of penis, dorsal and deep.

External Iliac Artery:

Begins at lumbo-sacral articulation from bifurcation of common iliac.

Ends at distal border of inguinal ligament by continuing as femoral.

Relations:

	Anterior.		*Posterior.*
Put	Peritoneum.	**Physicians**	Psoas muscle
In	Intestines.	**Frequently**	and its fascia.
The	Testicular vessels.	**Opened**	Obturator nerve.
Ureter	Ureter.	**Veins.**	External iliac
Near	Genito-femoral		vein.
	nerve.		
Vas	Vas deferens.		
Deferens.	Deep circumflex iliac		
	vein.		

Femoral Artery:

Begins as continuation of external iliac at distal border of inguinal ligament.

Ends at opening in the adductor magnus by becoming popliteal.

Relations:

(A) In Femoral Triangle.

	Anterior.		Posterior.
Surely	Skin.	**Femoral**	Femoral sheath.
Some	Sartorius.	**Vein**	Femoral vein.
Fascia	Fascia (superficial, deep).	**Passes**	Profunda vessels.
		Proximally	Pectineal fascia.
Makes	Medial cutaneous nerve.	**Near**	N. to pectineus.
		Psoas	Psoas.
Femoral	Femoral branch of genito-femoral nerve.	**Pectineus.**	Pectineus.
Sheath.	Femoral sheath.	**Add. Longus.**	Adductor longus.

Branches:

Skilful	Superficial epigastric.
Surgeons	Superficial circumflex iliac.
Should	Superficial external pudendal.
Detect	Deep external pudendal.

Gastric	Descending geniculate.
Perforations.	Profunda.

(B) In Subsartorial Canal.

Anterior.

Should	Skin.
Find	Fascia (superficial, deep).
Sartorius	Sartorius.
Placed	Subsartorial plexus.
Above	Aponeurotic roof.
Saphenous nerve.	Saphenous nerve.

Posterior.

Adductor	Adductor longus.
Muscles	Adductor magnus.
Flex.	Femoral vein.

Lateral.

Veins	Femoral vein.
Seldom	Saphenous nerve.
Not	Nerve to vastus medialis.
Variable.	Vastus medialis.

Profundal Femoris Artery :

Begins one and a half inches distal to the inguinal ligament as a branch of the femoral artery.

Ends perforating the adductor magnus as the 4th perforating artery.

Relations :

	Anterior.		*Posterior.*
Let	Adductor longus.	**I**	Iliacus.
Femoral	Femoral vein.	**Prefer**	Pectineus.
Pass.	Profunda vein.	**Brief**	Adductor brevis.
		MSS.	Adductor magnus.

Branches :

Let	Lateral circumflex
Most	Medial circumflex.
Men	Muscular.
Pass.	Perforating.

Popliteal Artery.

Begins as continuation of the femoral at the opening in the adductor magnus.

Ends at the distal edge of the popliteus by subdivision into (a) anterior tibial; (b) posterior tibial.

49

Relations:

	Superficial.		*Deep.*
Former	Fascia.	Free	Femur.
Conscientious	Post cutaneous nerve of thigh.	Parking	Posterior ligament of knee joint.
Students	Short saphenous vein.	Provided.	Popliteus and its fascia.
Make	Muscles bounding the space.		
Medical	Medial popliteal nerve.		
Practitioners.	Popliteal vein.		

Branches:

General Medical Council.	Geniculate. Muscular. Cutaneous.

D

Posterior Tibial Artery:

Begins at distal border of popliteus from bifurcation of popliteal.

Ends at distal border of flexor retinaculum of ankle by sub-division into medial and lateral plantars.

Relations :

	Superficial.		*Deep.*
Susie	Skin.	Timothy	Tibialis posterior.
Finds	Fascia and flexor retinaculum.	Does	Flex. digitorum longus.
Golfing	Gastrocnemius.	Take	Tibia (distal end).
Specially	Soleus.	Port.	Posterior ligament of ankle.
Promotes	Posterior tibial nerve.		
Health.	Abductor hallucis brevis.		

Branches :

Peroneal	Peroneal.
Muscles	Muscular.
Clearly	Cutaneous.
Notch	Nutrient to tibia.
Malleolus	Malleolar.
Contiguous	Communicating to peroneal.
Calcaneus	Medial calcanean.

Medial Plantar Artery:

Begins at distal border of flexor retinaculum from bifurcation of posterior tibial.

Ends by joining plantar digital artery to the medial side of great toe.

Branches :

D.	Digital.
C.	Cutaneous.
M.	Muscular.

Lateral Plantar Artery:

Begins at distal border of flexor retinaculum from posterior tibial.

Ends as plantar arch at base of 1st metatarsal by joining with dorsalis pedis.

Branches:

Medial	Muscular.
Calcanean	Medial calcanean.
Cutaneous	Cutaneous.
Partly	Perforating (to dorsal metacarpal arteries).
Plantar	Plantar metatarsal arteries (3).
Distribution.	Digital (to lateral side of little toe).

Anterior Tibial Artery:

Begins at the distal border of the popliteus from the bifurcation of the popliteal.

Ends at the distal border of the ankle joint by changing its name to dorsalis pedis.

Relations :

	Anterior.		*Posterior.*
The	Tibialis anterior.	**F.**	Front of ankle joint.
Fascial	Fascia.	**I.**	Interosseous membrane.
Retinaculum	Extensor retina-	**T.**	Front of tibia.
	culum.		
Holds	Extensor hallucis		
	longus.		
Down	Extensor digi-		
	torum longus.		
All	Anterior tibial		
	nerve.		
Structures.	Skin.		

Lateral.

H. Extensor hallucis longus.
A. Anterior tibial nerve.
D. Extensor digitorum longus.

Branches :

A	Anterior tibial recurrent.
Physican	Posterior tibial recurrent.
Can	Circumflex fibular.
Make	Muscular.
Cough	Cutaneous.
Mixtures.	Malleolar (lateral, medial).

Dorsalis Pedis :

Begins at distal border of ankle joint by continuation of anterior tibial artery.

Ends on plantar aspect of 1st metatarsal by joining lateral plantar artery.

Branches :

F.	First metatarsal (dorsal, plantar).
A.	Arcuate artery.
C.	Cutaneous.
T.	Tarsal.

NOTES

VEINS.

Note.—In general (1) Above the level of the diaphragm veins are superficial to their arteries. (2) Below level of diaphragm veins are deep to their arteries except (*a*) veins in the region of the kidney; (*b*) profunda femoris vein.

Internal Jugular Vein :

Begins at jugular foramen as the continuation of the sigmoid sinus.

Ends at the sternoclavicular joint by joining the subclavian to form the innominate vein.

Tributaries :

Faucial	Common facial.
Tonsils	Thyroid (superior, middle).
Lie	Lingual.
In	Inferior petrosal sinus.
Pharynx.	Pharyngeal.

Inferior Vena Cava :

Begins in front of the body of the 5th lumbar vertebra by union of the common iliac veins.

Ends—pierces diaphragm opposite 8th dorsal vertebra and ends piercing pericardium in lower and back part of right atrium.

Tributaries :

Portal	Phrenic. ⎫
System	Suprarenal. ⎬ Right.
Returns	Renal. ⎭
To	Testicular.
Liver	Lumbars (3rd and 4th).
In	Common iliacs.
Humans.	Hepatics.

Portal Vein :

Begins behind neck of pancreas by the union of splenic and superior mesenteric veins opposite 1st lumbar vertebra.

Ends at hilum of liver subdividing into right and left branches, each of which break up into capillaries around the liver lobules.

Derives blood from :

Should	Spleen.
George	Gallbladder.
Personally	Pancreas.
Purchase	Peritoneum.
Ladies'	Large ⎫ Intestines.
Silk	Small. ⎭
Stockings ?	Stomach.

NOTES

HEART.

Position of Valves :

1. Pulmonary.—Upper border of 3rd left costal cartilage at sternal junction.

2. Aortic.—Lower border of 3rd left costal cartilage behind left half of sternum.

3. Mitral.—Upper border of 4th left costal cartilage behind left half of sternum.

4. Tricuspid.—4th intercostal space behind right half of sternum.

N.B.—Thus openings are placed :

Pulmonary.	Upper border of 3rd	⎫
Aortic.	Lower border of 3rd	⎬ left costal cartilage.
Mitral.	Upper border of 4th	⎭
Tricuspid.	Lower border of 4th right costal cartilage.	

Points of interest in Right Atrium:

Some	Superior caval opening.
Inherit	Inferior caval opening.
Valuable	Valve of inferior vena cava.
Possessions	Musculi pectinati.
And	Atrio-ventricular opening.
Can	Opening of coronary sinus.
Find	Fossa ovalis.
Lucrative	Limbus ovalis.
Foreign	Foramen ovale.
Investments	Intervenous tubercle.
Constantly	Crista terminalis.
Available.	Anterior cardiac veins.

NERVOUS SYSTEM.

Exit of Cranial Nerves from Skull :

1st.	Olfactory.	Cribriform plate of ethmoid.
2nd.	Optic.	Optic foramen.
3rd.	Oculomotor.	
4th.	Trochlear.	} Superior orbital fissure.
5th.	Trigeminal (ophthalmic nerve).	
6th.	Abducens.	

5th. Trigeminal. { Maxillary nerve.—Foramen rotundum.
Mandibular nerve.—Foramen ovale.

7th.	Facial.	} Auditory meatus.
8th.	Auditory.	
9th.	Glossopharyngeal.	
10th.	Vagus.	} Jugular foramen.
11th.	Accessory.	
12th.	Hypoglossal.—Condyloid canal.	

Classification of Cranial Nerves:

Nerves of Special Sense.	*Motor Nerves.*	*Mixed Nerves.*
Olfactory.	Oculomotor.	Trigeminal.
Optic.	Trochlear.	Glossopharyngeal.
Auditory.	Abducens.	Vagus.
	Accessory.	
	Hypoglossal.	

Oculomotor Nerve.

Nucleus.—In anterior part of grey matter around cerebral aqueduct at the level of superior corpus quadrigeminum.

Point of Emergence.—Through the medial sulcus of the mid-brain.

Course.—(1) Through interpeduncular cistern with posterior cerebral artery above, superior cerebellar artery below, and posterior communicating artery medial.

(2) Pierces dura of the roof of the cavernous sinus lateral to the posterior clinoid between free and attached borders of the tentorium cerebelli.

(3) In the cavernous sinus lies the highest structure in the lateral wall, and then is crossed laterally from below upwards by the trochlear nerve. It divides into two branches.

(4) These pass through the superior orbital fissure into the orbit between the two heads of the lateral rectus and embracing the nasociliary nerve.

(5) The upper division distributes to the levator palpabrae and superior rectus.

(6) Lower division distributes to medial rectus, inferior rectus, inferior oblique and gives a motor root to the ciliary ganglion.

Course indicated by :

Through peduncular cistern first I run,
Then pierce dura—just for fun ;
Here posterior clinoid is to medium
Between the two borders of tentorium.
Next laterally in the sinus I go,
Crossed by trochlear from below ;
Into two branches then I split
And these round nasociliary fit.
Thro' orbital fissure next I pass
Between the heads of the lateral rectus,
Entering orbit that I may
Supply levator palpabrae.
Inferior oblique and recti three,
With twig to the ganglion come from me.

E

Trigeminal Nerve.

Branches of Ophthalmic Nerve :

Four	Frontal.
Lazy	Lacrimal.
Navvies	Nasociliary.
Don't	Dural.
Care.	Communicating to 3rd, 4th, 6th Sympathetic.

Branches of Maxillary Nerve :

Much	Meningeal.
Guinness	Ganglionic to spheno-palatine ganglion.
Zooms	Zygomatic.
Down	Dental (posterior, middle, anterior).
Past	Palpebral
Lips	Labial.
Nightly.	Nasal.

Branches of Mandibular Nerve :

Never	Nervus spinosus.	} TRUNK.
Make	Medial pterygoid nerve.	
Ladies	Lateral pterygoid nerve.	
Take	Temporal (anterior, posterior) deep.	} ANTERIOR DIVISION.
Beauty	Buccal.	
Massage.	Masseteric.	
Leave	Lingual.	
It	Inferior dental.	} POSTERIOR DIVISION.
Alone.	Auriculo-temporal.	

Facial Nerve.

Cortical nucleus.—In face centre of precentral gyrus.

Supranuclear Fibres :

Descend with the motor tract through the corona radiata knee-shaped bend of the internal capsule, medial part of the motor fibres of the pes, to decussate with their fellows and reach the opposite facial nucleus.

Nucleus. (1) **Motor nucleus.**—Lies deeply placed in lower pons dorsal to dorsal nucleus of corpus trapezoideum and deep to floor of the 4th ventricle distal to the superior fovea.

(2) **Sensory nucleus.**—Upper end of tractus solitarius of medulla.

Infranuclear Fibres :

(1) **Within pons.**—From nucleus fibres encircle abducens nucleus and pass down forwards and laterally joined by sensory root to

(2) **Point of emergence** at lower and lateral border of pons medial to auditory nerve in cerebello-pontine angle.

(3) **Enters skull** at internal auditory meatus with sensory root, auditory nerve and internal auditory artery below it. At lateral end of meatus incorporates sensory root, pierces dura and enters facial canal.

(4) **In facial canal** nerve runs—

Oh
Be
Damned !

(a) *Outwards* in roof of internal ear with cochlea in front and vestibule behind to gain medial wall of middle ear.

(b) *Backwards.*—Makes a knee-shaped bend—the genu—and passes backwards in substance of the medial wall of the middle ear above fenestra vestibuli and below lateral semicircular canal, to the aditus, where it turns

(c) *Downwards*—in the posterior wall of the middle ear and anterior to the sigmoid sinus to find

(5) **Exit from skull** at stylomastoid foramen. Thus commences

(6) **Cervical course,** where the nerve curls down and forwards, entering posterior and deep aspect of the parotid, crossing

(a) Styloid process ;
(b) Internal jugular ;
(c) Internal carotid ;
(d) External jugular ;
(e) External carotid ;
(f) Mandible ;

(7) **Reaching face** to subdivide into (a) Temporo-facial and (b) Cervico-facial, from which terminal branches pierce parotid fascia to reach the muscles of expression.

Gay	Great superficial petrosal — to sphenopalatine ganglion.	
Little	Root to lesser superficial petrosal —to otic ganglion.	In Temporal Bone.
Elves	External superficial petrosal—to middle meningeal.	
Stoop	Nerve to stapedius.	
To	Chorda tympani.	
All	Communicating to vagus.	
Dancing	Posterior auricular.	In Neck.
Sweetly.	Posterior belly of digastric.	
To	Stylohyoid.	
Useful	Temporal.	
Labour	Upper zygomatic.	
Bring	Lower zygomatic.	On Face.
Me	Buccal.	
Cautiously.	Mandibular.	
	Cervical.	

Glossopharyngeal Nerve.

Branches :

The	Tympanic nerve.
Physician	Pharyngeal branches.
Spots	N. to stylopharyngeus.
Large	Lingual.
Tonsills.	Tonsillar.

Vagus Nerve.

Branches :

Many	Meningeal.
A	Auricular.
Prodigal	Pharyngeal.
Son	Superior laryngeal (subdivides into internal and external).
Runs	Recurrent laryngeal.
Carelessly	Cardiac.
Through	Thoracic cardiac.
A	Anterior pulmonc

Of	Oesophageal.
Gold	Gastric.
Principally	Pancreatic.
In	Intestinal.
Sumptuous	Splenic.
Living.	Liver.

Hypoglossal Nerve.

Branches :	
Men	Meningeal.
Converse	Communicating to vagus and sympathetic.
Discretely	Descending—with descendens cervicalis forms ansa hypoglossi which innervates infrahyoid muscles. N. to thyrohyoid.
To	Lingual—geniohyoid,
Ladies.	genioglossus,
	styloglossus,
	hyoglossus,
	intrinsic muscles.

Gladly	
Giving	
Some	
Helpful	
Information.	

Phrenic Nerve.

Branches:

Do	Diaphragmatic.
Petting	Pleural.
Parties	Pericardial.
In	Inferior vena caval.
Private	Peritoneal.
Harm	Hepatic.
Anyone ?	Adrenal.

Brachial Plexus.

Lateral Cord.
Branches come
from C. 5 6 7.
{ Lateral pectoral.
Lateral head of median.
Musculo-cutaneous.

Medial Cord.
Branches come
from C. 8, D. 1.
{ Medial pectoral.
Medial cutaneous of arm.
Medial cutaneous of forearm.
Medial head of median.
Ulnar

DISTRIBUTE
TO FRONT
OF UPPER
LIMB.

Posterior Cord. {

Axillary C. 5 6.

Subscapular C. 5 6.

N. to lat. dorsi. C. 6 7 8.

Radial nerve C. 5 6 7 8 D. 1.

} DISTRIBUTE TO BACK OF UPPER LIMB.

Musculo-cutaneous Nerve.

Branches :

(1) Muscular to the 3 Bs.—biceps.
   brachialis.
   coracobrachialis.

(2) Lateral cutaneous of forearm.

Median Nerve.

Branches:

Assistants
Must
Articular.
Muscular to—
Pronator teres.
Flex. carpi radialis.
Palmaris longus.
Flex. digitorum sublimus.

Acquire
Anterior interosseous—
½ Flex. digitorum profundus.
Flex. poll. longus.
Pronator quadratus.

Proper
Palmar cutaneous.

that is:
All Muscles of Front of Forearm except (1) Flex. carpi ulnaris; (2) ½ Flex. digitorum profundus.

Medical
Diplomas.
Muscular to thumb.
Palmar digital—lateral 3½ digits.

In Palm:
L. LAT. 2 LUMBRICALS.
O. OPPONENS POLL.
A. ABD. POLL. BREVIS.
F. FLEX. BREV. POLL.

Ulnar Nerve.

Branches :

Artists'
Models

Articular to elbow.

Muscular to—Flex. carpi ulnaris.
½ Flex. digit. prof. } In Forearm.

Pose
And
Dull

Palmar cutaneous—to skin over hypothenar
eminence.

Articular—to wrist.

Dorsal cutaneous—to ulnar side of wrist, dorsum
and ulnar 1½ digits.

Students

Superficial division—to palmaris brevis and volar
aspect of ulnar 1½ digits.

Dip.

Deep division to—

Abductor digiti minimi.
Opponens digiti minimi.
Flex. digiti minimi.
All interossei.
Adductor obliquus poll.
Adductor transversus poll.
Medial 2 lumbricals.

All Short
Muscles
of Palm
except
L.
O.
A.
F.

Radial Nerve.

Branches :

Muscular to brachioradialis.
brachialis.
extensor carpi rad. longus.
anconeus.
triceps.

       "B.,"
       B.
       E.
       A.
       T.

Articular to elbow.

Cutaneous—Post. cut. of upper arm.
Lower lat. cut. of upper arm.
Post. cut. of forearm.
Terminal to—
   radial side of wrist.
   radial ⅔ of dorsum of hand.
   radial 3½ dorsal digits.

Put
Little
Finger
There.

Posterior interosseous—muscular to—

All Muscles on Back of Forearm *except* Bea of Beat.
$\left\{\begin{array}{l}\text{Extensor carpi rad. brevis.}\\\text{Extensor digitorum communis.}\\\text{Extensor digiti minimi.}\\\text{Extensor carpi ulnaris.}\\\text{Supinator.}\\\text{Abd. poll. long.}\\\text{Ext. poll. long.}\\\text{Ext. poll. brev.}\\\text{Ext. indices.}\end{array}\right.$

Lumbar Plexus.

Lies in substance of psoas. Nerves emerge from margins of the psoas.

		EMERGE FROM PSOAS.
I	Iliohypogastric T. 12, L. 1.	LAT. SIDE.
Invariably	Ilioinguinal T. 12, L.1.	
Let	Lateral cutaneous L. 2 3.	
Flo	Femoral, L. 2 3 4.	ANT. SURFACE.
Go	Genito-femoral, L. 1 2.	
Out.	Obturator, L. 2 3 4.	MEDIAL SIDE.

Obturator Nerve.

Branches :

Some	Articular to sacroiliac joint.	TRUNK.
Husbands	Articular to hip joint.	
Perhaps	Pectineus.	
Like	Adductor longus.	ANTERIOR DIVISION.
Good	Adductor gracilis.	
Beer.	Adductor brevis.	
Some	To subsartorial plexus.	
Are	Vascreator to femoral artery

Adductor brevis (sometimes).
Obturator externus.
Articular to knee.
Adductor magnus. } POSTERIOR DIVISION.

Femoral Nerve.

Branches:

Better — N. to iliacus.
Educated, — Vasomotor to femoral artery. } FROM TRUNK IN PELVIS.

Accumulating —
Money. —

I — N. to pectineus.
Find — Medial cutaneous.
Psoas — Intermediate cutaneous.
Muscle — N. to sartorius. } FROM SUPERFICIAL DIVISION.

Is —
Sometimes —

Quite — Nerves to quadriceps extensor—
    Rectus femoris.
    Vastus lateralis.
    Vastus intermedius.
    Vastus medialis. } DEEP DIVISION.

Small. — Saphenous nerve.

IN FEMORAL TRIANGLE.

Sacral and Coccygeal Plexus.

1 nerve comes by **5** roots—sciatic L. 45, S. 1 2 3.
4 nerves come by **2** roots.
6 nerves come by **3** roots.

4 Nerves by 2 roots:

Queer N. to quadratus femoris from lumbo-sacral cord and 1 S.

People N. to pyriformis, S. 1 2.

Enjoy Nervi erigentes, S. 2 3.

Anatomy. Nerves to anal muscles—coccygeus. levator ani. ext. sphincter. $\left.\right\}$ S. 3 4.

6 Nerves by 3 roots:

So Superior gluteal N., L. 45, S. 1.

I opine. $\left\{\begin{array}{l}\text{Inferior gluteal;} \\ \text{N. to obturator internus.}\end{array}\right\}$ L. 5, S. 1 2.

Sacral Small sciatic (post. femoral cut.), S. 1 2 3.

Plexus Pudendal, S. 2 3 4.

Not *None from* S. 3 4 5.

Simple. Sacrococcygeal S. 4 5, C. 1.

NOTES

Sciatic Nerve.

Branches :

Hamstrings	Articular to hip joint.
Always	Adductor magnus.
Supplied	Semimembranosus.
By	Biceps.
Sciatic.	Semitendinosus.

Origin L. 45, S. 123 is within pelvis. Leaves pelvis through greater sciatic foramen.

Termination at upper apex of popliteal fossa by subdivision into medial and lateral popliteal.

Relations outside Pelvis :

	Superficial.
Get	Gluteus maximus.
Powder	Pyriformis.
Box.	Long head of biceps.

	Medial.
Tie	Tuber ischii.
My	Semimembranosus.
Tie.	Semitendinosus.

	Deep.
A	Acetabulum (post. lip).
Nerve	N. to quad. femoris.
Goes	Gemelli.
Into	Obturator internus.
Fossa	Quad. femoris.
Of	Obturator externus.
Acetabulum.	Adductor magnus.

	Lateral.
Tie	Great trochanter.
My	Gluteus maximus (insertion).
Bonnet.	Short head of biceps.

Lateral Popliteal Nerve:

Origin as the smaller terminal branch of the sciatic at upper apex of popliteal fossa.

Termination winding round lateral side of neck of fibula in substance of peroneus longus to subdivide into anterior tibial and musculo-cutaneous.

Course lies on	**From**	
	Patella	Femur (post. surface).
	Goes	Plantaris.
	Supra-	Gastrocnemius (lat. head).
	Patellar	Soleus.
	Pouch.	Popliteus.
		Peroneus longus.

Branches :

Let's	Lateral cutaneous nerve of calf.
Swallow	Sural communicating.
Glucose	Geniculate lateral (superior, inferior).
And	Ant. tibial.
Make	Musculo-cutaneous.
Records.	Recurrent geniculate.

Anterior Tibial Nerve :

Origin from bifurcation of lateral popliteal in the substance of the peroneus longus.

Termination at distal border of extensor retinacula subdivides into medial and lateral branches.

Branches :

Timothy	Tibialis anterior.
Has	Extensor hallucis longus.
Done	Extensor digitorum (longus, brevis).
Trixie	Peroneus tertius.
Dirt.	1st digital cleft (dorsum).

Musculo-cutaneous Nerve:

Origin from bifurcation of lateral popliteal in the substance of the peroneus longus.

Termination in cutaneous distribution on the dorsum of the foot.

Branches :

Let	Peroneus longus.
Britain	Peroneus brevis.
Conquer.	Cutaneous to distal third of leg.
	dorsum of foot.
	all dorsum of toes except 1st digital cleft.

Medial Popliteal:

Origin larger terminal branch of the sciatic at upper apex of popliteal fossa.

Termination at distal edge of popliteus by changing its name to posterior tibial.

Branches :

Get   Medial geniculate—superior.
middle.
inferior.

Some Sural nerve.
G.Ps. Gastrocnemius.
Plantaris. } Muscular branches.
Popliteus.
Soleus.

Posterior Tibial Nerve:

Origin as continuation of medial popliteal as distal edge of popliteus.

Termination by subdivision into medial and lateral plantars under cover of distal third of flexor retinaculum.

Branches :

So	Soleus.
Timothy	Tibialis posterior.
Has	Flex. hallucis longus.
Done	Flex. digitorum longus.
A	Articular to ankle.
Comic	Median calcanean.
Tango.	Terminal— medial plantar.
	lateral plantar.

Medial Plantar Nerve.

Branches :

D. Digital to plantar aspect medial 3½ toes.

C. Cutaneous to medial side of sole.

M. Muscular to—abductor hallucis.

flex. brev. digitorum.

flex. brev. hallucis.

1st lumbrical.

} All other Short Muscles of Sole are by Lat. Plantar.

The Medial Plantar Nerve supplies

The Abd. Hall. 'neath which it lies.

The Flexor Brev. Dig. and Hall.

And Lieber Gott! 1st Lumbrical!

Lateral Plantar Nerve.

Branches :

D. Digital to plantar aspect lateral 1½ toes.

C. Cutaneous to lateral side of sole.

M. Muscular to (1) Flexor accessorius ;

(2) Abductor digiti minimi ;

(3) Flex. digiti minimi brevis ;

(4) Adductor hallucis brevis ;

(5) Lateral three lumbricals ;

(6) All interossei.

Structures passing through Superior Orbital Fissure.

Lie practically on the same plane and enter the orbit above the lateral rectus, to lie between the roof of the orbit and the orbital muscles.

(1) **Two**	Trochlear.	
(2) **Fat**	Frontal N.	From
(3) **Ladies**	Lachrymal N.	Ophthalmic N.

Lie below the above (1), (2) and (3), entering the orbit between the two heads of the lateral rectus in numerical order from above down and from lateral to medial.

(4) **Supping**	Superior division of oculomotor.
(5) **Nice**	Nasociliary from ophthalmic N.
(6) **Ices**	Inferior division of oculomotor.
(7) **Are**	Abducens nerve.
(8) **Vanished.**	Ophthalmic veins.

Structures passing through the Cavernous Sinus.

From above downward :

Offers	Oculomotor N.	
To	Trochlear N.	IN
Operate	Ophthalmic N. of trigeminal.	LATERAL WALL.
Are	Abducens N.	IN
Cautiously	Internal carotid artery.	MEDIAL WALL.
Made.	Maxillary N. of trigeminal.	IN LATERAL ANGLE.

Structures passing through Foramen Ovale.

Men	Mandibular N. (motor, sensory) of trigeminal.
Like	Lesser superficial petrosal nerve.
An	Accessory meningeal artery.
Energetic	Emissary vein.
Lady.	Meningeal lymphatics.

Structures passing through Foramen Magnum.

Spinal	Spinal cord.
Meninges	Spinal meninges.
Make	Meningeal lymphatics.
A	Accessory nerves (spinal roots).
Special	Sympathetic plexus on vertebral arteries.
Vertical	Vertebral arteries.
Sheath.	Spinal branches of vertebral arteries.

Structures passing through Greater Sciatic Foramen.

Please	Posterior femoral cutaneous nerve.	
Note	N. to quadratus femoris.	
I	Inferior gluteal vessels and nerve.	BELOW
Pass	Pudendal nerve.	PYRIFORMIS.
No	N. to obturator internus.	
Students	Sciatic nerve.	
In	Internal pudendal vessels.	

Second Superior gluteal vessels and nerve. } PYRIFORMIS.
Professional. Pyriformis muscle.

Structures passing through **Lesser Sciatic Foramen.**

Not N. to obturator internus.
To-night, Tendon of obturator internus.
Please! Pudendal vessels and nerve.

Innervation of Extrinsic Muscles of Eye.

(1) Levator palpabrae. ⎫
(2) Superior rectus. ⎪ By oculomotor N.
(3) Inferior rectus. ⎬ *thus note* (**L.R.₆S.O.₄**)₃.
(4) Medial rectus. ⎪
(5) Inferior oblique. ⎭
(6) Superior oblique—by trochlear N.
(7) Lateral rectus—by abducens N.

Layers of the Scalp.

S. Skin.
C. Close connective tissue and cutaneous vessels and nerves.
A. Epicranial aponeurosis.
L. Loose connective tissue.
P. Pericranium.

Digastric or Submandibular Triangle.

Boundaries :

SUPERIORLY.—(1) Mandible ; (2) An imaginary line from its angle to the tip of the mastoid process.

POSTERO-INFERIORLY.—(1) Posterior belly of digastric ; (2) Body of hyoid bone.

ANTERIORLY.—Midline of neck from symphysis menti to hyoid bone.

FLOOR.—(1) Mylohyoid ; (2) Hyoglossus ; (3) Middle constrictor.

ROOF.—(1) Skin ; (2) Superficial fascia ; (3) Platysma muscle; (4) Deep fascia.

Contents :

Do	Anterior belly of digastric.
Not	N. to mylohyoid. ⎫
All	Artery to mylohyoid. ⎬ From inf. dental.
Glands	Submandibular gland. ⎭
Have	Hypoglossal nerve.
Some	Stylomandibular ligament.
Protective	Parotid gland (portion of).
Fascial	Facial vessels.
Covering?	External carotid art. giving off posterior auricular.

G

Carotid Triangle.

Boundaries :

ANTERO-SUPERIORLY.—(1) Posterior belly of digastric ; (2) Stylohyoid.

ANTERO-INFERIORLY.—Superior belly of omohyoid.

POSTERIOR.—Sternomastoid.

ROOF.—Skin, superficial fascia, platysma, muscle and deep fascia.

FLOOR.—(1) Hyoglossus ; } Anteriorly.
      (2) Hyoid bone ; }

      (3) Thyrohyoid ;
      (4) Thyrohyoid membrane ; } Posteriorly.
      (5) Middle constrictor ; }
      (6) Inferior constrictor.

Contents :

A. Arteries :

    (1) Common carotid.
    (2) Internal carotid.
    (3) External carotid with branches :
        (a) Superior thyroid ;
        (b) Lingual ;

    (c) Facial;

    (d) Occipital;

    (e) Ascending pharyngeal.

B. Veins:

Internal jugular, receiving tributaries :

    (a) Superior thyroid ;

    (b) Lingual;

    (c) Common facial;

    (d) Pharyngeal ;

    (e) Communication from external jugular.

C. Nerves :

  (1) Vagus and branches :

    (a) Internal laryngeal;

    (b) External laryngeal.

  (2) Accessory.

  (3) Hypoglossal and branches :

    (a) Descendens hypoglossi ;

    (b) N. to thyrohyoid.

  (4) Sympathetic.

D. Other Structures :

  (1) Carotid body.

  (2) Anterior superior deep cervical lymph nodes.

Subclavian Triangle.

Boundaries :

POSTERO-SUPERIOR.—Inferior belly of omohyoid.

ANTERIOR.—Sternomastoid.

INFERIOR.—Clavicle (middle third).

FLOOR.—(1) Scalenus medius; (2) Scalenus anterior (sometimes); (3) 1st digitation of serratus anterior; (4) 1st rib.

ROOF—(1) Skin; (2) Superficial fascia; (3) Platysma muscle; (4) Supraclavicular nerves; (5) Deep fascia.

Contents :

S. Subclavian artery 3rd part and subclavian vein (sometimes).

T. Transverse cervical artery.

E. External jugular veins and tributaries—(anterior jugular, transverse cervical, suprascapular).

N. N. to subclavius.

T. Trunks of the brachial plexus.

S. Suprascapular artery and nerve.

Axilla is a pyramidal-shaped space between upper part of chest wall and upper arm. Not a perfect pyramid because (1) Apex is truncated; (2) Posterior wall is longer than anterior; (3) Medial wall is broader than lateral. Axillary shape is maintained under all circumstances because of (1) Crossing of fibres of pectoralis major; (2) Twisting of fibres of latissimus dorsi; (3) Attachment of clavicle to axillary base by clavi-pectoral fascia.

Boundaries:

ANTERIOR WALL.—(1) Clavicle; (2) Subclavius; (3) Pectoralis minor; (4) Clavi-pectoral fascia; (5) Pectoralis major.

POSTERIOR WALL.—(1) Scapula; (2) Subscapularis; (3) Latissimus dorsi; (4) Teres major.

MEDIAL WALL.—(1) Upper five ribs; (2) Corresponding interior-costal spaces; (3) Corresponding digitations of serratus anterior.

LATERAL WALL.—(1) Coracoid process; (2) Head, neck and upper part of shaft of humerus; (3) Coracobrachialis and short head of biceps.

BASE.—Axillary fascia.

APEX.—The cervico-axillary canal, bounded (1) Anteriorly by clavicle; (2) Posteriorly by upper border of scapula; (3) Medially by 1st rib.

Contents :

Birmingham	Brachial plexus—infraclavicular part and its branches.
Nomenclature	N. to serratus anterior.
Lately	Lymph nodes.
Introduced	Intercosto-brachial nerve.
Vastly	Axillary vein and its tributaries, *N.B.* Cephalic v.
Improves	Lateral cutaneous branches of intercostal nerves 3 and 4.
Anatomy.	Axillary artery and its branches.

Cubital Fossa is a triangular fossa in front of the elbow.

Boundaries :

BASE.—An imaginary line taken between the two epicondyles.

LATERALLY.—Brachioradialis.

MEDIALLY.—Pronator teres.

APEX.—Crossing of brachioradialis over pronator teres.

ROOF.—(1) Skin; (2) Superficial fascia containing (3) Median cubital vein; (4) Lateral cutaneous nerve; (5) and Medial cutaneous nerve of forearm; (6) Deep fascia with bicipital aponeurosis.

FLOOR.—Brachialis—above and medially. Supinator—below and laterally.

Contents :

T. Tendon of the biceps.
A. Brachial artery subdividing into (1) radial; (2) ulnar.
N. Median nerve.

Flexor Retinaculum at Wrist.—Is a thick, strong, fascial band bridging the carpal groove, converting it into a carpal tunnel. It is continuously proximally with the deep fascia of the forearm and distally with the palmar aponeurosis.

Attachments:

Radial $\left\{\begin{array}{l} \textbf{S.} \\ \textbf{T.} \\ \textbf{O.} \\ \textbf{P.} \end{array}\right.$

Ulnar

Tubercle of Scaphoid.
Groove on Trapezium.
Hook of Os' Hamatum
Pisiform.

Order of Structures at Proximal Border of Flexor Retinaculum.

From Superficial to Deep.

(1) Skin.
(2) Superficial fascia with—

$\left.\begin{array}{l} \text{(a) Lateral cutaneous nerve of forearm ;} \\ \text{(b) Palmar cutaneous branch of median ;} \\ \text{(c) Palmaris longus ;} \\ \text{(d) Palmar cutaneous branch of ulnar.} \end{array}\right\}$ *Order from Radial to Ulnar Side.*

(3) Superficial part of retinaculum (volar carpal ligament).

—Deep Fascia—— becoming—— Flexor Retinaculum—

Order from Radial to Ulnar Side.

(4) Extensor pollicis brevis.
Abductor pollicis longus.
Superficial palmar branch of the radial artery.
Flexor carpi radialis.
Median nerve.
Flexor sublimus—tendons to middle and ring fingers.

Ulnar vessels ⎱ thence proceed distally superficial to flexor retinaculum but
Ulnar nerve ⎰ deep to superficial part of retinaculum.

Flexor carpi ulnaris.

(5) Flexor pollicis longus.

(6) Flexor sublimus—tendons to index and little fingers.
Flexor profundus—two tendons, viz.: (a) one separate for index; (b) one common to medial three digits.

(7) Recurrent branches of the deep palmar arch.

Order of Structures in the Hollow of the Palm.

(1) Skin.

(2) Superficial fascia—intersected by fascial bands connecting skin to deep fascia—with palmar cutaneous branches of median and ulnar nerves.

(3) Palmar aponeurosis.

(4) Superficial arch.

(5) Median and superficial division of ulnar nerves.

(6) Flexor digitorum sublimus tendons } enclosed in

(7) Flexor digitorum profundus tendons } synovial sheath— with lumbricals } ulnar bursa.

(8) Deep division of ulnar nerve.

(9) Deep palmar arch.

(10) Adductor pollicis brevis, interossei muscles and meta- carpal bones.

Thus, by putting an IMAGINARY plane between flex. sublimus and profundus, we get—

Palmar Aponeurosis.
Superficial Arch.
Median Nerve.
Flex. Sublimus.

--------- IMAGINARY PLANE ---------

Flex. Profundus.
Ulnar N. (Deep Division).
Deep Arch.
Bones and Interossei Muscles.

A muscle in front and a muscle behind,
A nerve in front and a nerve behind,
An artery in front and an artery behind,
Fascia in front and bones behind.

But *N.B.*—that digital branches of superficial arch pass deep to digital branches of median and ulnar nerves.

Short Muscles of Hand and Foot.

Thumb.	Little Finger.	Great Toe.	Little Toe.
Abductor (Poll. Brev.) Adductor. Flex. Brevis. Opponens.	Abductor (Digiti Minimi). No ADDUCTOR. Flex. Brevis. Opponens.	Abductor (Hall Brevis). Adductor. Flex. Brevis. No OPPONENS.	Abductor (Digiti Minimi). No ADDUCTOR. Flex. Brevis. No OPPONENS.

All insert into appropriate medial or lateral side base of 1st phalanx, except the (1) Opponens pollicis—main insertion radial side of metacarpal of thumb ; (2) Opponens digiti minimi—main insertion ulnar side of metacarpal of little finger.

Interossei Muscles.

(A) Of Hand.—Are **8** in number, viz. : (1) **4** palmar ; (2) **4** dorsal. ACTION.—(1) Palmar interossei adduct. and dorsal interossei abduct.—in relation to the middle finger (longest finger). (2) All the interossei also flex the metacarpo-phalangeal and extend the interphalangeal joints.

INSERTION.—(1) 1st palmar interosseous inserts into ulnar side base proximal phalanx of thumb. (2) All the rest insert into (a) the extensor tendon; (b) base of proximal phalanx; (c) capsule of metacarpo-phalangeal joint.

ORIGIN.—(1) Palmar interossei come from the palmar aspect of the metacarpal of the digit on which they act. (2) Dorsal interossei come from the dorsal aspect of the contiguous sides of the metacarpals between which they lie.

POSITION.—Thus *palmar interossei are arranged* fulfilling origins and insertions as above—

    1st on ulnar side of thumb,
    2nd on ulnar side of index finger,
    3rd on radial side of ring finger,
    4th on radial side of little finger.

And dorsal interossei are arranged—

    1st on radial side of index finger,
    2nd on radial side of middle finger,
    3rd on ulnar side of middle finger,
    4th on ulnar side of ring finger.

NERVE SUPPLY.—All interossei of hand are supplied by *deep division of ulnar nerve.*

Interossei Muscles—*continued.*

(B) Of Foot.—Interossei are **7** in number—**3** plantar (which ad-duct,) and **4** dorsal (which abduct.)—in relation to 2nd toe (longest toe). Their other actions, origins and insertions correspond to that fellow of the hand.

PLANTAR INTEROSSEI are arranged on tibial side of 3rd, 4th and 5th toes.

DORSAL INTEROSSEI are arranged 1st on tibial side of 2nd toe, 2nd, 3rd and 4th on fibular sides of 2nd, 3rd and 4th toes.

NERVE SUPPLY.—All interossei of foot are supplied by lateral plantar N.

Thus middle finger receives **2** dorsal but no palmar; 2nd toe receives **2** dorsal but no plantar.

2 middle finger, 2 second toe
That for the dorsal ones, Yo ho !
None middle finger, none second toe
That for the palm and plantars go.

NOTES

Extensor Retinaculum of Wrist.—Is a thickened portion of the deep fascia on the back of the forearm. It is weaker, longer, more proximal than the flexor retinaculum and in direction is oblique from radial to ulnar side. It is attached laterally to the distal end of the radius in the margin between anterior and lateral surfaces, and medially to triquetrum, pisiform and flexor retinaculum, and deeply by **5** septae to the margins of the grooves on the dorsal aspects of radius and ulna, converting them into six fibro-osseous canals for the transmission of the extensor tendon and their synovial sheaths.

Attachments of Extensor Retinaculum.

R. Radius—ridge lateral to pronator quadratus.
U. Ulna.
P. Pisiform.
T. Triquetrum.

Fibro-osseous Compartments, Extensor Tendons and Synovial Membranes beneath Extensor Retinaculum.

		RADIUS	ULNA
A Beautiful	Abd. poll. long. Ext. poll. brev.	1 synov. memb. Groove lat. side distal end of radius.	
Little Bride	Ext. carpi. rad. long. Ext. carpi. rad. brev.	1 synov. memb. Groove dorsal-ulnar to radial styloid.	
Looks	Ext. poll. long.	1 synov. memb. Oblique groove medial to dorsal tubercle of radius (Lister's tubercle).	
Distressed If	Ext. digitorum Ext. indices.	1 synov. memb. Most medial groove on dorsal aspect of radius.	
Minus	Ext. dig. minimi.	1 synov. memb. *Groove between radius and ulna.*	
Undies.	Ext. carpi ulnaris.		1 synov. memb. Groove between ulnar styloid and head of ulna.

H

Structures covered by the Gluteus Maximus.

A. 1 LIGAMENT—

The sacro-tuberous ligament.

B. 2 BONY POINTS—

(1) Tuber ischii ;

(2) Great trochanter.

C. 3 BURSAE—

(1) Over tuber ischii ;

(2) Between gluteus medius insertion and great trochanter ;

(3) Between gluteus maximus and vastus lateralis.

D. 6 VESSELS—

(1) Superior gluteal vessels ;

(2) Inferior gluteal vessels ;

(3) Internal pudendal vessels ;

(4) Medial circumflex (ascending, transverse) branches ;

(5) Lateral circumflex—transverse branch ;

(6) 1st perforating branch of profunda femoris.

E. 7 Nerves—

(1) Superior gluteal nerve ;
(2) Inferior gluteal nerve ;
(3) Sciatic nerve ;
(4) Posterior femoral cutaneous N. ;
(5) N. to quadratus femoris ;
(6) N. to obturator internus ;
(7) Pudendal nerve.

F. 8 Muscles—

(1) Gluteus medius ;
(2) Pyriformis ;
(3) Obturator internus and gemelli ;
(4) Obturator externus tendon ;
(5) Quadratus femoris ;
(6) Adductor magnus ;
(7) Origin of the hamstrings ;
(8) Vastus lateralis.

Cutaneous Nerves of Gluteal Region.

S. Sacral nerves.— {Perforating cut. of S. 2 and 3 (ant. rami).
Cutaneous brs. of S. 1, 2 and 3 (post. rami).

L. Lumbar nerves—cut. brs. of L. 1 2 3 (post. rami).
I. Iliohypogastric—lat. cut. br.
D. 12th dorsal N. (subcostal) lat. cut. br.
E. Ext. (lat.) cutaneous n. of thigh—post. branch.
S. Small sciatic n. (post. femoral cutaneous)—recurrent brs.

Femoral Triangle.—Is a superficial triangular space in the proximal third of the anterior surface of the thigh.

Boundaries :

BASE.—Inguinal ligament.

APEX.—Crossing of sartorius over the adductor longus.

LATERAL.—Medial border of sartorius.

MEDIAL.—Medial border of adductor longus.

ROOF.—Fascia lata and cribriform fascia.

FLOOR.—Is furrow-shaped, having iliopsoas laterally; and pectineus, adductor brevis (sometimes), and adductor longus medially.

Contents :

S. Femoral sheath.

C. Femoral canal—medial compartment of sheath.

A. Femoral artery and its branches—superficial epigastric ;
circumflex iliac ;
ext. pudendal ;
profunda.

V. Femoral vein and its tributaries—saphenous ;
circumflex ;
deep ext. pudendal ;
profunda.

A. Ant. division of obturator N. (if brevis forms floor).

N. Femoral N. and its branches.

G. Femoral branch of genito-femoral nerve.

E. External (lat.) cutaneous N. of thigh.

Subsartorial Canal.—Is an intermuscular canal on the antero-medial aspect of the middle third of the thigh, extending from the apex of the femoral triangle proximally to the opening in the adductor magnus distally.

Boundaries:

ANTERO-MEDIAL.—(1) Sartorius; (2) Aponeurotic fascia extending between vastus medialis and the adductor longus and magnus.

ANTERO-LATERAL.—Vastus medialis.

POSTERO-LATERAL.—(1) Adductor longus; (2) Adductor magnus.

Contents:

A	Femoral artery.
Good	Its descending geniculate branch.
Valet	Femoral vein.
Should	Saphenous N.
Never	N. to vastus medialis.
Laugh.	Deep lymphatics.

The **Popliteal Fossa** is a diamond-shaped space at the back of the knee.

Boundaries :

SUPERO-LATERAL.—Biceps.

SUPERO-MEDIAL. — Semimembranosus and semitendinosus — supplemented by gracilis, sartorius and adductor magnus.

INFERO-LATERAL.—Plantaris and lateral head of gastrocnemius.

INFERO-MEDIAL.—Medial head of gastrocnemius.

FLOOR.—Popliteal surface of the femur. } Proximal
Posterior ligament of the knee joint. } to
Popliteus muscle and its fascia. } Distal.

ROOF.—Skin, superficial fascia with posterior femoral cutaneous nerve and short saphenous vein, popliteal fascia.

Contents :

A Popliteal artery and its branches—cutaneous ; muscular ; genicular (5).

Vain Popliteal vein and its tributaries—corresponding to arterial branches ; short saphenous.

Man Medial popliteal N. and its branches.

Greatly Geniculate branch of the obturator nerve.

Likes Lateral popliteal N. and its branches.

Loud Lymph nodes.

Praise. Post. femoral cutaneous nerve.

Note.—In Femoral Triangle ⎱ the relative positions of artery,
Subsartorial Canal ⎰ vein and nerve are indicated by
and Popliteal Fossa remembering

(1) (a) When the sartorius muscle is lateral (to the artery) the
vein is medial (to the artery)—Femoral Triangle.

(b) When the sartorius is superficial the vein is deep—
Subsartorial Canal.

(c) When the sartorius is medial the vein is lateral—
proximal end of Popliteal Fossa.

(2) All nerves crossing arteries in the lower extremity do so
superficially from lateral to medial side (in the position
of dissection)—except the posterior tibial (which crosses
its artery superficially from medial to lateral side).

Retinaculae at the Ankle.—In the region of the ankle the deep fascia is thickened into bands binding down the tendons that pass in relation to the ankle and forming compartments usually with synovial linings for their transmission. There are recognised—

(1) Extensor Retinaculum :

(a) SUPERIOR.—Between distal parts of anterior border of tibia and fibula binds bellies of muscles of leg. 1 synov. memb. for tibialis anterior.

(b) INFERIOR.—Y-shaped. Stem on lateral side at junction of anterior, superior and lateral surfaces of calcaneus. Limbs on medial side—proximal to medial malleolus, distal to fascia on medial side of foot. Binds tendons to dorsum of foot. 3 synov. membs. for tibialis anterior, ext. hallucis longus, ext. digitorum longus and peroneus tertius.

(2) Flexor Retinaculum :

Extends from medial malleolus to medial tubercle of calcaneus.

3 synov. membs. for tibialis posterior, flexor digitorum longus, and flexor hallucis longus.

(3) Peroneal Retinaculae :

(a) SUPERIOR.—Holds peroneal tendons to back of lateral malleolus. 1 synov. memb.

(b) INFERIOR.—Binds peroneal tendons to lateral side of calcaneous. Space is split by a septum attaching to peroneal tubercle. 2 synov. membs. for peroneus longus and peroneus brevis.

Arrangement of Structures beneath Retinaculae at Ankle.

Timothy	Tibialis anterior.	
Hath	Extensor hallucis longus.	
Vexed	Vein.	
All	Ant. tibial artery.	BENEATH
Very	Vein.	EXTENSOR
Nervous	Ant. tibial nerve.	RETINACULUM
Dairymaids	Extensor digitorum longus.	FROM MEDIAL
Through	Peroneus tertius.	TO LATERAL.
Flirting.	Fibula.	
Timothy	Tibialis posterior.	
Doth	Flexor digitorum longus.	
Vex	Vein.	BENEATH
All	Post. tibial artery.	FLEXOR
Very	Vein.	RETINACULUM
Nervous	Post. tibial nerve.	FROM MEDIAL
Housemaids.	Flexor hallucis longus.	TO LATERAL.

Bad
Lad.

Peroneus brevis.
Peroneus longus.

BENEATH PERONEAL RETINACULAE
FROM—(1) BEFORE BACK AT LAT.
MALLEOLUS; (2) ABOVE DOWN ON
CALCANEUS.

FROM CALCANEUS.

Layers of Sole of Foot.

(1) Deep fascia and plantar aponeurosis.

SHORT MUSCLES.

(2) Abductor hallucis—from (a) flex. retinaculum; (b) medial tubercle of calcaneus.
Flex. digitorum brev.—from medial tubercle of calcaneus.
Abductor digiti minimi—from medial and lateral tubercles of calcaneus.

LONG MUSCLES.

(3) Flexor accessorius—from (a) long plantar lig.; (b) plantar surface of calcaneus; (c) medial surface of calcaneus.
Flex. hallucis longus.
Flex. digitorum longus and lumbricals.

(4) Adductor hallucis.

SHORT MUSCLES.

Transverse head.—from (a) plantar surface of deep transverse ligament; (b) plantar ligs. of lat. 4 metatarsophalangeal joints.

Oblique head—from (a) sheath of peroneus longus; (b) bases of 2nd, 3rd, 4th metatarsals.

Flex. brev. hallucis—from (a) medial aspect of plantar surface of cuboid; (b) tib. post. slips to lat. and middle cuneiforms.

Flex. digiti. minimi brevis—from (a) sheath of peroneus longus; (b) plantar surface of 5th metatarsal base.

(5) LONG MUSCLES. Tendon of tibialis posterior.
Tendon of peroneus longus.

(6) SHORT MUSCLES. Interossei.

Order of Structures in Parotid Gland.

No Facial N.
Villains Origin of external jugular vein.
Allowed. External carotid artery.

Contents of Carotid Sheath.

Idleness Internal jugular vein—lateral.
Causes Carotid artery (internal, common)—medial.
Vice. Vagus N.—post. and between.

Root of Lung.

Components :

(1) Pulmonary artery.
(2) Two pulmonary veins.
(3) Bronchus.
(4) Bronchial art. and veins.
(5) Hilus nodes and pulmonary lymphatics.
(6) Pulmonary nerve plexuses.

RELATIVE POSITIONS OF MAIN COMPONENTS?

FROM ABOVE DOWN—

	Left Side.		*Right Side.*
Are	Pulmonary artery.	**Brides**	Eparterial bronchus.
Brides	Bronchus.	**Are**	Pulmonary artery.
Vain?	Lower pulmonary vein.	**Beastly**	Hyparterial bronchus.
		Vain.	Lower pulmonary vein.

FROM BEFORE BACK :

Verily	Upper pulmonary vein.
Are	Pulmonary artery.
Brides !	Bronchus.

Structures at Hilum of Kidney.

FROM BEFORE BACK :

V.	Renal vein.
A.	Renal artery.
D.	Duct (ureter).

Structures at Hilum of Liver.

FROM BEFORE BACK :

D. Hepatic ducts. ⎫
A. Hepatic arteries. ⎬ Right and Left.
V. Portal veins. ⎭

Note.—The general arrangement at the hilum of organs is—

(1) Vein. ⎫
(2) Artery ⎬ from before back,
(3) Duct ⎭

but in the liver developmental rotation reversed this order.

POSITION AND RELATION OF KIDNEYS.

Each kidney is a bean-shaped organ $\begin{cases} 4\frac{1}{2} \text{ inches long.} \\ 2\frac{1}{2} \text{ inches broad.} \\ 1\frac{1}{4} \text{ inches thick.} \end{cases}$

It lies in retroperitoneal position in the paravertebral recess, obliquely placed so that the upper pole is nearer to the middle line, and bulkier, its lateral surface looking forwards and laterally. It is opposite the 12th rib and the first three lumbar vertebrae, the right kidney reaching upper border of the 12th rib and the left to the lower margin of the 11th. The lower pole is just supraumbilical and a little above the top of the iliac crest at the level of the subcostal plane (3rd L.V.). Transpyloric plane cuts middle of left hilum 2 inches from middle line.

Anterior Relations :

	Right Kidney.		*Left Kidney.*
Superiorly	Suprarenal.	**8 Ss.**—Suprarenal.	
Duodenum	2nd part of duodenum.		Spleen.
			Splenic vessels.
Adjoins	Rt. colic art. (ascending br.).		Splenic ligaments.
			Splenic flexure (left colic) or transverse colon.
Liver	Liver.		Stomach.
Peritoneum	Peritoneum.		Small intestine.
Fixing	Rt. colic flexure.		Sweetbread (pancreas).
Intestine.	Small intestine.		

Posterior Relations :

DIRECT RELATIONS :

1 Artery—
Subcostal artery.

2 Bones—
(1) 12th rib ;
(2) Transverse processes of 1st three lumbar vertebrae.

(1) Subcostal ;
(2) Iliohypogastric;
(3) Ilio-inguinal.

4 Muscles and their fascia—

(1) Psoas ;
(2) Quadratus lumborum ;
(3) Transversus ;
(4) Diaphragm.

First the diaphragm I see,
Then three muscles P.Q.T. ;
Three nerves* with I for their initial,
The first and second lumbar vessel,
Three vertebrae across it run,
12th rib and ligaments arcuatum,
Vertebro-costal trigone on occasion,
And the pleura as an indirect relation.

---

* The third nerve is subcostal = "last intercostal"—anatomical licence !

NOTES

NOTES